A Gift To

Me

From

Me

Date

1-10-0L

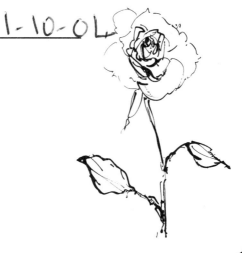

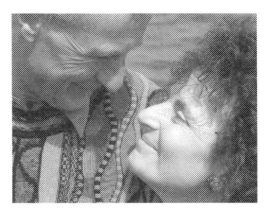

Roger and Linda King

MEDITATIONS & AFFIRMATIONS ON
MAKING LOVE WITH
PASSIONATE
THOUGHTS

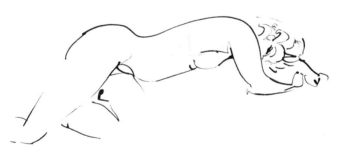

BY ROGER KING

Linda,
with so much
love, Roger.
xxx

Also by Roger King
'Love the Miracle You Are'

First published in 2004 by Soul Talk Stories.
3 Waterton Close, Walton, Wakefield, West Yorkshire WF2 6JT, UK.
Email Roger at roger@soultalkstories.com and visit the website www.soultalkstories.com

The moral right of the author has been asserted.
Cover art and Illustrations by Linda King ©Copyright 2004.

Printed in England by Harris Brothers, Pontefract, West Yorkshire.

My affirmation for this soul talk book No 2 is

I marvel at the possibility of making love every moment of every day, by breathing abundant air that lovingly supports the miracle of my life!

The more I come from a place of deep respectful love in my soul, the more I will love our creator, my neighbour and my self.
And so it is.

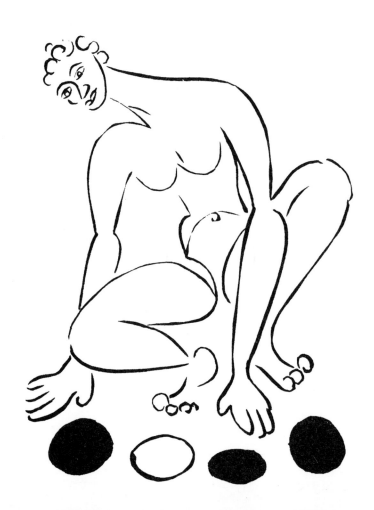

This little book is dedicated to all who are on the journey of the "way" that is being increasingly travelled to raise our consciousness of divine energy.

PREFACE TO THIS FIRST EDITION

It is a year since I wrote *"Love The Miracle You Are."*

I am deeply moved by the feedback on how that book is touching people's lives of all backgrounds. I would like to thank the wonderful team around me, including John Welding, illustrator. Paul Armitage, business adviser, Chelle Thompson, editor, Vidya Ishaya, web designer and Karin Peterson-Sitrin personal coach. I thank also my family and friends. Having taken a leap of faith 6 months ago to self-publish, after many rejections, the rewards have been a steep learning curve with hard work; yet the 'inner voice' has kept me on track with increasing love, purpose and meaning. I affirm this second 'Soul Talk Stories' book will help you get on track to your "Way" and give your mind, body and soul a sustenance that is given by 'loving thoughts.'

Roger King
2004

Please note our website is www.soultalkstories.com and we welcome your stories that come from your soul. We will be publishing some of the stories on the website in future paperback books, one called "Breaking Free To Love," with the aim of spreading your love around our world to help heal our planet.

WHY THIS BOOK?

The simple aim of this book is to develop our 'higher awareness' by feeding our unconscious mind positive messages, from our conscious mind. This I believe helps each of us experience our lives with intimacy and compassion, as unique and responsible human beings, with our lives working and manifesting our destiny, to bring healing and peace to this planet. Making love with passionate thoughts helps us to grow positively from the years of pain.

What it is NOT is a shallow positive book that masks our pain or looks down on others who are in pain. We often come to our lives as a victim feeling powerless; consequently making our lives even more painful by the energy we put out, by the thoughts we think and say from the limiting belief patterns that we hold (learned by 3 to 7 years old).

Making love with passionate thoughts will help heal your mind because you give yourself permission to choose thoughts that don't side step pain, yet transform your pain into a higher awareness. This starts and continues your day with a love of yourself, connected to a loving, healing universal mind and to other souls who are thinking healing thoughts. I believe each of us has a soul that is divinely guided and protected. We are not just our pain with fragmented lonely thoughts of fear, anger and criticism. When I awake and lie in bed, I can so easily sabotage my day with old, sluggish negative thoughts that block my higher awareness, where I stay in the past and recreate the past as though it is my present.

By persistently reading and saying aloud these "Affirmations & Meditations on Making Love with Passionate Thoughts," you will gradually change your energy from self-defeating, draining thoughts that originate in the lower self, to a deep self-respecting love that nurtures our higher self. The inner child was told so often with negative passion "you're not good enough." This can leave us feeling a victim, depressed and addicted to blaming. We carry these old messages within us … and they are lies.

To undo these lies and dissolve them takes time and patience. When you repeat positive affirmations over and over again, you will notice positive changes within and around you. These are thoughts you would love to know are true, yet at first you will doubt them, because they appear not to be true. For example *"I love and approve of all of me, even the blind spots!"* may seem like a foreign language.

Making love from a higher awareness develops our creative inner imaginative child; these thoughts attract joy and inner freedom, which allow you to learn from both good and tough experiences to embrace the paradoxes of life.

• From higher self-thinking on learning to love ourselves as a miracle, we ignite a spark that seeks all good. We come to every experience with a vision of new possibilities and live in the now, which allows us to have tears from our pain, yet know we will move on and NOT stay a victim.

• By saying positive, loving thoughts to your self, you will build a deep core of trust in your mind, body and soul.

Your intuition will gradually dissolve the thoughts of threat and the need for constant approval from others.

• Your inner child will feel freer to think and act with a "spontaneous intelligence."

• You will embrace the uncertainties of life, as you live life now.

By saying and believing compassionate thoughts like *"I choose to make love with passionate, positive thoughts from my conscious mind, repeated often to my unconscious mind; this helps me accept me just as I am. And so it is."* This simple message reveals a beauty that heals our soul and cannot deny the miracle of our life.

No matter how sceptical you are at first, the 'Cosmic Mind' that made us notices when you say loving thoughts from your conscious mind to your unconscious mind; and the law of what you put out comes back with such love and forgiveness that this in turn creates joy! To talk with loving intelligence to the miracle power within us is a challenge to you and me in a world that can seem so unjust.

THE POWER OF AFFRIMATIONS

Affirmations are anything that we think and say. Our thoughts create our feelings, beliefs and experiences. So often, they are negative. So often we say, "I hate my life" or "I am no good at relationships." If we truly want to change and grow, we need to see the old limiting thoughts and feelings as LIES that we believed from those around us. Then we can give up the need to blame and begin to state what we DO want with positive passion and compassion for others, including ourselves.

Affirmations that say, " I forgive you" do not deny your old family patterns of negative beliefs or the well of tears or the inequalities, yet they allow you to see and let go the pain you carry and let love become larger than any need to continue expressing your experience from a place of being a victim. Affirmations empower you the more you use them, ESPECIALLY when your reality says they are NOT true.

By repeating these affirmations as daily meditations you are preparing yourself for the climb of your spiritual, mental and physical life. As I make love —not war, in my life: "I am open and receptive to all good and I let go, with love, any old needs for self-criticism, fear and guilt." This little book comes with my everyday experiences and enthusiasm of using these bite-size meditations. I hope you keep it handy; flick through and wherever it opens, perhaps that's the meditation most appropriate for you at the time.

Remember, nothing exists in the past, it happens always in the now. The 'lower self' comes from your old subconscious mind that picked up messages of 'never being good enough.' Whenever you come from these old negative beliefs and messages, you can feel the energy drain from you, your power goes and you blame everyone including yourself. This is the alchemy of life, to choose and say thoughts that bring life into being in the moment of now. This is where God meets the road in your thought, speech and your moment-to-moment action! And so it is.

MEDITATION 1. POWER OF THE MIND

*"The spirit cannot be, or become antagonistic towards us. It is always
flowing into us and ever expressing itself through us..."*
Ernest Holmes, The Science of Mind

Our Thoughts are so powerful in creating and shaping our experiences in life, so
say with passion and arms out wide:

*I am open and receptive to all good
and I make love with every moment
of life. I see and think more clearly
with love.*

To allow in "all good" dissolves the old message "I deserve a good smack!"
To sit quietly and slow your thoughts each day is like washing your body in a crystal
clear pool of clean mountain water. For me there is a thrill of being in the presence of
that universal mind that says: *"I love you and I will never harm you, even
when life gets tough."*

MEDITATION 2. CONSCIOUS MIND

"What was wonderful to learn was that the thoughts I chose to think determined my experiences from moment-to-moment. Then what I put out from my mind came back multiplied in experience."

Roger

The conscious mind is self-knowing, self-assertive, it has will, choice and may accept or reject. It is the only part of our mind that can think independently of circumstances, affirm consciously:

When I say, "Yes" to life, the universal mind notices and gives me more healing and vigorous energy. This is the dynamic law of what I put out comes back multiplied with interest.

MEDITATION 3. UNIVERSAL & SUB-CONSCIOUS MIND

*"The sub-conscious mind is simply the Law of Mind in action.
It is not a thing of itself but is the medium for all thought action. It is the
medium by which man may call into temporary being whatever he needs
or enjoys on the pathway of his experience."*
Ernest Holmes, The Science of Mind

I believe when life gets tough the universal mind is showing us a mirror to see and understand a lesson that we may choose to learn from or carry on until it hurts us time and time again. So to make passionate and positive present tense thoughts from our conscious mind to our sub-conscious mind is an incredible gift of love to ourselves and all to whom we connect, affirm:

Everything works out for my highest good, even when life appears tough. I know, for myself, that every thought I am thinking in the present creates my present and future reality. And so it is.

MEDITATION 4. MAKING LOVE

Is a natural gift of life, like breathing; it brings the elements of the invisible into the visible and back to invisible by starting a creative and miraculous cycle of life. Most of us may think of the physical act of loving another person that stirs our fantasies and appetite for pleasure. What a gift, when used well and from a place of love within each of us; yet there are so many more ways we can make love in this human temple. Each of us has so much love to give and receive. Learning to come from the tears of joy puts us in contact with a love so rich and real that our hearts burst into the song of our souls, affirm:

> *I make love with my mind, body and spirit and this creates love with passion.*

Witnessing a baby's birth, watching a sunset with deep gratitude, cooking and serving a beautiful meal are ways of giving from our higher self. Making love is listening to somebody's life story … where their unique path and talent are saying "yes" from a place that reveals their truth moment by moment. Making love with passionate thoughts is being awakened by the whisper of the universal mind that prompts you to prayer or meditation in the middle of the night.

It is about walking gently with God's soul whispering thoughts that manifest all good in you, where you see and think outside the tramlines of your past and the dogma of old beliefs. Making love with passionate thoughts is about risking appearing a fool by going beyond fashion and negative news; it is diving deeper to find the current of life that moves with love, where new souls will swim with us. We may never meet them in this life, but know them through thought, an email friendship, or a soul glance on a crowded street.

MEDITATION 5. DREAM

Often dreams get knocked out of us at an early age, yet I dare you to dream the dream that lays dormant in all of us, that is the miracle to love and be loved with passion. During the day or week you may have a dream, a thought or an experience that reveals the process, or clue, or possibly an answer. Again affirm the following:

> *I give myself permission to go beyond others and my own limitations and I am constantly redefining who I am and how I want to live. I grow to love and forgive others, and myself, a little more.*
> *And so it is.*

When you have a negative thought like "I am too fat" or "too thin," just experiment by asking "What do you really think and feel?" Then shut your eyes and go within to a quiet meditation and ask:

"What is it I need to know?"
"What is it I need to learn?"
"What do I have to give?"

MEDITATION 6. LOVE YOUR SELF AND LET GO OF THE NEED TO CHANGE OTHERS

As a counsellor I realised after many years of trying to change others that I could not help anybody unless they were willing to change and grow, to know this was such a relief. To begin to accept that all good is NORMAL for you is a divine gift from the universal mind. You cannot force this good upon anybody else. Just send love … remember you have your lessons, I have mine, affirm:

I love myself in such a way that lets go of the need to change others; the only person I can change is me. As I learn to love me, all parts of me, the more I set myself free to radiate unconditional love to all whom I meet. And so it is.

MEDITATION 7. LOVE YOUR INNER CHILD

"Come to me like a child and the kingdom of heaven is yours."
Jesus

Creating a loving inner parent nurtures the inner child that you have been criticising too long, the more you release the genius of your inner child and inner teenager the more your adult can live in the present with wonder, creativity and joy! All thoughts are affirmations, so I choose to think and say positive thoughts to my inner child, affirm with passion.

> *I love you, inner child, and I want to enjoy your trust in me. I let go of any need to hurt you. I love you unconditionally.*
> *And so it is.*

Your inner child has been scolded enough; let it out to play with your positive inner parent. Read John Bradshaw's The Home Coming and John Pollard's Self-Parenting. These two books will help your passion for living with an inner parent that says, "I love you, little child, come to me and I love you with new insights that set us free to become true friends."

Say this into a mirror as often as you remember — and just notice!

MEDITATION 8. CHALLENGE CONFORMITY WITHOUT BLAME

"Whoso would be a man, must be a non-conformist. He who would gather immortal palms must not be hindered by the name of goodness, but must explore if it be goodness. Nothing is at last sacred but the integrity of your own mind."

Ralph Waldo Emerson, An Essay on Self-Reliance

You and I are not our mother's or father's fears, criticisms and beliefs. Those who continue to blame will never become self-reliant in an empowered way. Each of us can dilute old limiting and erroneous beliefs by acting "AS IF" — then believing, by consistently repeating the following thought passionately affirm:

I now choose to think thoughts that are fresh, creative and loving. I use my own mind to learn and flow without blame of others and myself.
And so it is.

Wherever you are now, write your own affirmations … as many as you can. There is a universal magic that comes when you write and say out loud your positive thoughts in your self-reliant mind.

MEDITATION 9. FORGIVING

"Forgiveness recognises what you thought your brother did to you has not occurred"

A Course In Miracles

I awoke this morning with excitement and this affirmation formed in my mind.

> *I radiate love as I learn to let go of the past by forgiving all who hurt me, including myself. I release the past with positive insight and go within where I find new strength to grow and change my consciousness. And so it is.*

Leading my life with my wounds was a hard journey; often my pain was the only deep feeling I thought I could express to the world with any degree of authenticity. Having a positive loving life seemed miles away from my reality. This did not help to attract other loving souls; I seemed to attract to me more hurting, angry and guilty souls. Yet this was part of my journey. Now I see how I can change the quality of my life by consistently choosing to go beyond my old thought and feeling patterns. I am not denying my scars from old wounds, yet I now give conscious forgiveness to those who made those wounds, from a deeper soul consciousness that is expanding and setting us all free. And now I begin to give sincere thanks.

MEDITATION 10. JOY

"Joy and ecstasy come from within ... they cannot be bought at any price."
Roger

As a rather intense or serious person I have wanted to "lighten up!" My old Buddhist teacher would shout "Lighten up, Roger, the room lights up when you leave it!" This hurt my inner child yet there was a truth in this and I hated to hear it. My hate did not help me to hear his love for me, affirm:

I now accept that there is an infinite well of joy and ecstasy deep at the centre of my existence.

I am open and receptive to this abundant joy that fills my heart, my mind, my body and my conscious thought.
And so it is.

MEDITATION 11. CREATE BELIEFS THAT SUPPORT YOU

"What you give out comes back to you, what you believe about yourself and about life becomes true for you."

Louise Hay, Life!

Limitations of criticism, fear, guilt and resentment are old beliefs and habits of thinking that have gone into and around the subconscious mind for years. When I get up in the morning, I can so easily think and do the same functional thoughts. Yet when I get on my spiritual and mental bike, and get momentum by peddling conscious thoughts that give thanks for being alive, it's like the universal mind is immediately there with me.

I at once notice a shift in energy. Like now at 5 am, I am writing and I just feel great to be with the silence of creation. I look out and into my life with new meaning. When you wake up, repeat this affirmation with a passion; do it in front of the mirror … the universe notices!

> *When I make mistakes I say to myself, "I love you just as you are and I have the ability to turn each mistake into a lesson of growth and change. And I give thanks."*

Today I had the privilege of owning a mistake I made when I did not truly hear somebody in a counselling session. As I owned up to this, it immediately took us both to a deeper place of love and compassion. I learned that to "own" my mistake could be rich with insights and positive growth for all involved. We were open to seeing old belief patterns that did not serve either of us, it was a very rich time.

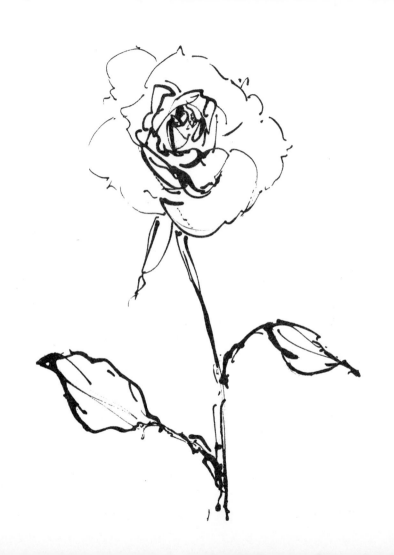

MEDITATION 12. GIVING & ATTRACTING

"The measure of mental health is the disposition to find good everywhere."

Ralph Waldo Emerson

Affirm:

> *I radiate to others what
> I want to receive and I choose
> to think, see, hear and be a channel
> for love, joy, creativity, forgiveness
> and fun. And so it is.*

When you are outside just notice people going about their lives and send love from your soul to them. I think of soul as the core that runs through the centre of my being and comes out through the top of my head … and is then joined to the energy source of all life. 'Smile LOVE' from deep within your soul at everyone you meet and see what comes back. You are not denying the pain in people's lives as you pass them in the street; you are offering new seeds of life. Wherever you go, see the opportunity to give love from the eternal well of love that is within you.

MEDITATION 13. DROP ALL CRITICISM, AND ACCEPT YOU JUST AS YOU ARE

"Once you accept that life is tough you can accept yourself just as you are and then the changes you make are so much more enjoyable and rich with coincidences and insights. The changes are good even when tough!" Roger

Affirm:

> # *I let go of all need to criticise others and myself. I choose to love and accept myself exactly as I am. And so it is.*

This is one of the most powerful affirmations that you or I can make in our lives. It is an invisible law that when I stop all criticism of others and myself, I move on to knowing:

"I am loveable, loving and loved because I exist."

Then I begin to make positive changes in my own life. I begin to see I can think thoughts that support my life and not beat me up. Life is tough enough without our continually criticizing ourselves, this just adds to life being hard. Make a passionate vow to stop all criticism. When you do criticise, just notice the thought and let it go with love.

MEDITATION 14. INNER POWER CREATES ENERGY

"The more I seek other people's approval all the time, the more I feel dominated and leak my true power of being powerfully loving, loveable and loved."   Roger

As we grow we will see old beliefs more clearly for what they truly are. They have served a purpose, yet some old beliefs now impede our growth. Our seeds of positive thoughts, repeatedly said with passion, give us an inner energy to move rocks of fear and pull out weeds of self-hatred and criticism. Remember, your subconscious mind cannot take a joke. It has recorded everything said and done to you and then repeated by you. Giving it loving thoughts will dissolve the pain and limiting beliefs. The more you send those positive thoughts with passion, the deeper the healing of old diseased thoughts that are hurting you.

Beliefs are thoughts and feelings that have become ingrained in our subconscious mind as "true". We learned these thought and feeling patterns from parents, teachers, lovers and misguided friends, and many people who were doing the best with what they knew. Learning to love yourself will allow you to let go of this erroneous need for other people's approval. Know for yourself:

I cannot afford the luxury of others' negative thoughts about me, their negative thoughts are not me. I release them with love. And so it is.

MEDITATION 15. PATTERNS

"Suffering is man-made, through ignorance....Someday we shall decide that we have had enough suffering"

Ernest Holmes, The Science of Mind

Affirm:

> *I choose loving thoughts to support my life now and in the future.*
> *And so it is.*

As I thought this I remember that I wanted to say, **"You are kidding yourself there's too much pain from your past to think like that."** This critical thought came from old-patterned thinking of feeling less intelligent than others when I was a child and teenager. This old, lower self-thinking does not allow love and healing energy to flow in or around me. So just sit and meditate on:

I choose positive, imaginative thoughts and they determine my experiences. I prosper in all areas of my life, in time, work, health, money, relationships and joy. I attract people in my life who respect me and I let go of old patterned thinking with love of those who hurt me.

MEDITATION 16. THE FLOW OF LIFE

"Everyone is coping with their past and present damaging patterns of old anger and fear. When I feel fear from the past, I can lose any sense of my present accomplishments. Then I can leak my power to love and forgive. I become blind to seeing; if I go within, I can renew my inner wisdom, especially when life gets tough." Roger

Within you are all the answers to all the questions you will ever ask. I can create my dark stormy clouds in my thoughts by criticising others or myself. The clouds thicken, and then I can be afraid of life and feel tossed like driftwood on a vast sea of despondency. Here I remember the affirmation:

I am at one with the flow of life; all life loves and supports me. And so it is.

Yes all life loves and supports us; when I am down that feels so foreign, yet it is true. Guideline: put your hands on your heart and repeat the above affirmation with passion.

MEDITATION 17. PERSONAL POWER

"Choose to see yourself as a unique individual not as a problem. You can grow as an individual, but seeing yourself as a problem leaks your personal worth and you join to other souls who see and think of themselves as problems." Roger

Becoming happy in life and work is learning to "choose" instead of thinking "I have to!" So often we can prove ourselves to be right and unhappy. For example *"I hate my job, I will never find a job that I like!"*

Take back your personal power by choosing a job you love, with an income that continuously increases and with people you like and who respect you.

Affirm:

> *I am open and receptive to a job that I love and I attract to me now a great job with people who love and value me, with an income that continues to increase.*

This creates a slightly different ring in the doorbell of life. If your reality is the opposite, begin thinking: *"I release my present job with love and allow a new job or career to manifest. And so it is."*

MEDITATION 18. HIGHER POWER

"We are each channels of thought that a great power operates through. The more we let this creative power work through us the more our consciousness attracts all good. We cannot coerce it; yet learning to love ourselves and others unconditionally, we become an increasingly clear channel for this higher power to work through us."

Roger

The more I start my day with meditation the more I sense this power that is there for me. It is like a force that slows me down to resonate with its infinite intelligence. I then get a glimpse of this higher power.

We rush to harness electricity, convert wind power, trap steam and use technology, yet with quiet simple meditation there is infinite power to tap residing within us, affirm with passion:

I now accept and become open to a power that has my highest good at the centre of its intention. I find deeply fulfilling ways to improve my life and I attract people who are in harmony with me. They accept me and we help each other from our higher power.

When any part of your life is not working, create a positive, present tense affirmation. *"I am connected to divine love, a higher power that is all love, the more I love me as a miracle of life, the more I connect to loving my life. And so it is."*

MEDITATION 19. GOOD ENOUGH

*"Have you never noticed that after you've shown a little love to someone,
a great wave of contentment pervades your entire being?"*
Osho, Sex Matters

I have a friend, Steve, who is a great teacher and author of children's books; each time we meet I sense his love and pain mixed with such humorous passion. We hug and know something of each other's love and pain without speaking of it. Our love for each other goes beyond barriers of "he's right and I am wrong," we just share with passion. I love sharing with people who are passionate about life because they are real givers. As you learn to love the miracle power within and around you, the more true friends will ignite laughter and tears from deep inside your soul; I give thanks for such soul friends on this planet. Real friends know a lot of your blind spots, yet accept you in a love that affirms the thought:

I am good enough just as I am.

*I attract great friends
who love me just as I am.
And so it is.*

Acceptance by another, even when you disagree, is like nectar to the soul.

MEDITATION 20. BLAME

"The more I learn to let go of blame, the more I sense and know a loving infinite intelligence that is there for me and you. Blaming is an act that keeps me in victim mentality and never lets me heal, it keeps creating the past hurt as though it is present hurt." Roger

Finding our treasures within and taking back our power by choosing to take responsibility for our lives, means letting go of all blame. This connects us to a divine energy that is always working for our highest good. So often, we can go through life attracting to us people and a concept of God that we can blame. It is like driving a car looking in the rear view mirror and wondering why we crash! When we stop all criticism and blame, we go within and feel connected to a source of all love. This abundant source is my experience of God, affirm:

I let go of all need to blame and criticise others or myself and this dissolves all barriers that delay my good and the channel of love that I can radiate to others.

And so it is.

MEDITATION 21. INSPIRATION

"When I feel inspired by some great purpose, all my thoughts break their past conditioning; my mind transcends my old limitations, and I see a wonderful energy make everything connected to a divine order."   Roger

We can go through life hoping we are going to win the lottery or football pools… I have won £10! When I always look for something OUTSIDE me to make me happy, I stumble. Yet it is different when I truly cry from deep within my soul and affirm this with arms wide open:

> *I am open and allow my soul to go beyond my fears. I go within and find the blueprint of divine love that goes beyond all of my old beliefs and feelings, and I give thanks.*

This calls into existence a power that directs us to revitalize dormant life. Instead of blaming, we see lessons to be learned from our previous life; all previous relationships take on a totally different meaning. We begin to see, hear, understand and get flashes of inspiration that touch an ancient wisdom of love and truth. From this place of going beyond the visible, we enter a beautiful garden where flowers grow and trees blossom. Increasingly we will attract all that we need to know at exactly the right time and in the perfect space sequence. It is not that we become greater in an egotistical sense, we become OPEN and RECEPTIVE to all good. So often a person will say, "I want to change my life, I am so unhappy!" I believe that by learning to love the miracle power within, we vision God's dream or blueprint for us.

MEDIATION 22. EMPOWERED CHILD

"Releasing with love the need to think of yourself as a victim, releases healing thoughts and words that change your experiences of life from hate to love." Roger

I love to be with my grandson and my children, yet at one time I found the demands of children so difficult, because I sensed I was a hurt child who was parenting them. I just had an emotional void that felt drowned in a sea of negative and unmet needs. I felt so much a victim blaming and wanting to be rescued; yet if anybody got close, I thought they would reject me if they got to know me. I became addicted to sex, and I hated myself.

As I learned to release my need for hating myself, I opened myself to a person who loved me. This brought up old resistances with many storms, yet as I accepted their love and started a deeper inner journey, I began to go within. I learned to accept myself and not beat myself up with thoughts of criticism, like "I am not good enough." I started to think, feel and affirm:

> *I love myself enough to love my frightened inner child, who has been scolded too long by my inner parent that was doing the best it knew how with what it knew.*

Many of us were parented by souls that didn't know why or how to love; they were doing the best with what they knew. I love seeing my inner child think and speak inside myself with an inner parent that loves and listens to that inner child. I now love my outer parents and forgive them; this one act has set me free to be me … all parts of me.

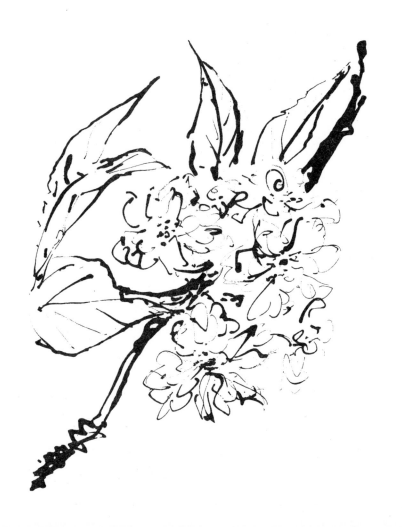

MEDITATION 23. INNER TALK

"I enjoy loving my inner child with a loving and forgiving inner parent; my inner self talk supports me now."

Roger

Thinking and saying inner child positive affirmations has released the 'wonder child' back into my life. This is the child that got lost in critical and resentful thoughts from parents, teachers and others, which I then carried inside my head as I grew into adult.

As I write this in my study, I look up and see all the inner child affirmations that started me writing. For example "I am willing to be patient with myself when I get off centre, I allow my inner parent to comfort me in my tears." Loving your inner child allows you to have intimate relationships with others. When we don't have any friends it is often due to an inner conversation that is so critical of your inner child, affirm:

I listen to my inner child each day and ask while looking into a mirror, "How can I help you feel loved and happy today?" Then I listen, and know I am there for them, and life takes on a whole new energy. We have fun creating life together, my child, my parent and my adult!

<u>MEDITATION 24. DESERVING GOOD</u>

"You will decide on a matter and it will be established
for you, and light will shine on your ways."

Job 22: 28

M aking a decision to deserve all good in your life is so foreign to the opposing thought "I don't deserve anything" or "I deserve a good smack" that it seems second nature to say to ourselves that we are not worthy … for this is not our first nature. If we learn this belief early as little children through religions, schools and parents, we then move through our life creating experiences to match our beliefs. Give yourself a chance to examine your thoughts of "not deserving good" and affirm *"I deserve joy, I deserve good in my life."*

Begin right now to think and say affirmations into a mirror:

I deserve all good, I deserve love and I deserve to be prosperous in all areas of my life. I am powerfully open and receptive to "deserving good things" back into my life right now. And I give thanks.

Change thoughts from "not deserving" to "deserving." You are worth it and the light will shine on your path.

MEDITATION 25. ORDERING FROM THE 'COSMIC CHEF'

"What we are today comes from our thoughts of yesterday, and our present thoughts build our life of tomorrow: our life is the creation of our mind."

The Buddha

When we push away our 'deserving good' by saying often inside our head, "I don't believe it" whenever something good happens to us, we are literally rejecting good in our lives.

Remember YOU choose the thoughts in your mind … nobody else; so by accepting good and giving thanks before and when you receive your good, you are opening yourself to even more abundant good from the "cosmic chef!" The cosmic chef is always listening to your inner self-talk, the orders you are giving yourself. Like "I can't do" … which is such an instruction to the power and presence in you to confirm "you can't." Watch carefully what you're saying to yourself and others, your inner and outer words are so powerful in creating your reality.

As I awake to ordering from the "Universal kitchen" with positive thoughts my present life hums with increasing meaning and purpose and the "cosmic chef" delivers exactly what I need at exactly the right time.

This order to the "cosmic chef" is such a powerful gift of love to your maker in the kitchen of the infinite universe.

MEDITATION 26. MEANING & PURPOSE

*"Our sense of meaning is the knowledge that we can truly
make a difference and that we are needed; we're important and that our
lives count for something. When we act in ways that are consistent with the
knowledge that we truly DO make a difference, our meaning and purpose
become clearer and our lives work on every level."*

Roger

To take back your power by ceasing to blame, and going quietly within each day, gives you a sense of a loving presence in your mind, heart and soul. This power gives meaning and purpose with intuitive regularity so that new meaning and purpose will pop in. Watch what a gift the universal mind will give you!

Affirm:

*As I love and accept myself a
new meaning and purpose reveals my
talent with new work, relationships
and a new path.*

And so it is.

MEDITATION 27. RELATIONSHIPS

" I now accept the perfect mate."

Louise Hay, Life!

As I talked to a lovely woman journalist who did a wonderful article on my first book, she said, "I am looking for a great partner can you find one for me?". As though somehow I could magically conjure up the person. She then read the little book called "Love The Miracle You Are" and today gave me a hug saying, "I have just attracted to me a lovely man." Then added "I also gave your book to my mum for Christmas and she said, 'It was my best present!'" Love radiates and heals. To love yourself from a place of deep self-respect is the best way to attract to yourself a partner who has the qualities YOU are creating in YOU. No one can ever love you enough if you don't love yourself, affirm:

> *My heart is open. I am now open and receptive to love flowing freely within me. As I love myself from a place of deep respect, I love others and the qualities I am creating in me attract exactly the right partner.*

Write down all the qualities you want in your partner, and then see if you're creating those in yourself. Stand in front of the mirror every day and say as often as you remember: *"Divine love is now leading me to, and maintains me in, a loving relationship with my perfect partner. And so it is."*

MEDITATION 28. PATIENCE WITHIN

"The more I go within each day in quiet
meditation the more I find wisdom, power
and the strength of patient love."   Roger

As we grow we may feel frightened to go within because we think we will find terrible things about ourselves! Yet whatever "they" have said about us, what you will find, as you meditate, will be a beautiful child that longs for love. The three, seven, forty and eighty year old child may be angry, silent and rebellious, yet crying out to be loved in every way.

As you move through the layers of other people's opinions and old beliefs you will heal, so affirm:

It is safe to go within
and hear the inner wisdom that
is there for me. I source from within
what I always wanted and needed
as a mind, body and soul to
feel complete.

And so it is.

MEDITATION 29. SEXUALITY

*"My sexual past no longer determines my
sexual experiences now."* Roger

I now rejoice in my sexuality! At one time my past thoughts of guilt and shame around my sexuality attracted to me similar partners. The outcome was often disastrous. Yet as I learned to love ME, I found such a beautiful woman, my present partner, who loved me as a whole person. When my past was my past, it no longer invaded me.

Affirm:

*I rejoice in my sexuality
and in my body.*

*This body is perfect for me and
I nourish it with loving thoughts,
nutritious food and I make love
and exercise with joy.*

And so it is.

MEDITATION 30. PASSIONATE THOUGHTS

The process of creating our own reality always requires strong and powerful thoughts, which come from a clear intention and a passionate desire. For much of my life I did not want to be a man, as I hated my own masculinity, body and men generally. Not a healthy belief system for anyone!

If you put your heart and soul into something, affirm these thoughts with passion! Say them with your arms open wide; when the resistance comes up, just thank it for sharing and carry on. As you say these affirmations you may feel they are untrue. They may not be true now; however, you can make them become true. Visualize, create mental scenes of you being these affirmations. We have so often used our imagination to create negative scenarios, now make a vow to make these positive, present tense affirmations true for you.

> *I am a strong and powerful miracle.*
> *I am intelligent and resourceful.*
> *I enjoy my sexuality.*
> *I am decisive.*
> *I am good at expressing myself.*
> *I continually increase my prosperity.*
> *I can think and see clearly in my mind.*

MEDITATION 31. CONNECTED TO NATURE

"As a counsellor I sometimes walk with clients through fields and woods as they unfold their pain. At times we stop and we hug trees and we sense the power of a tree to be a tree. It is such a gift to know nature knows how to be itself. This miracle of life is in you; it is waiting for you to discover the untried forces that are for your highest good. When you are in nature just look with your inner power and resonate with the wisdom and creativity of a blade of grass, or a rose, or a tree. Remember an acorn can only be an oak if planted in soil with all the right elements. Giving love to you is letting you receive all the right elements so you can become you."   Roger

Just notice what power resides in every living entity. I love ploughed fields, the tilled soil makes love with a passion that dance with my soul and I affirm with outstretched arms.

I am fully open and receptive to abundant wisdom in learning from nature. I see and think with vital energy that connects me to nature. And so it is.

MEDITATION 32. OPEN & RECEPTIVE

*"Change is a part of life and takes part in making us who we are.
When something we do not like happens to us, we have two options: to
become a bitter person or to become a better person."*

Marion Bond West, Motivational Author

"Pull yourself together and just get on with life, isn't it selfish to love yourself?" This was said to me on a radio interview. The interviewer was saying what he thought others would say to my book "Love The Miracle You Are". I replied "as we learn to love ourselves and feel really good enough to deserve all good, we will give love and radiate to others from abundance; rather than out of scarcity where we give out of guilt. When we give from guilt we radiate and attract blame and fear."

He carried on with "When you meet the real world, won't all this loving yourself go out the window?"My answer is simple "we create a false world of negativity when we are frightened of change and growth, where we stay stuck in anger, self-hatred, guilt and fear."Affirm with arms open and legs uncrossed.

*I am open and receptive
to all good that guides me to
my highest good and I radiate
this to the world.
And so it is.*

MEDITATION 33. DIVINE MOMENTS

"'Everything arises and passes away' when you see this, you are above sorrow. This is the shining way."

The Dhammapada, The Sayings of the Buddha

Today I arose feeling inspired by thoughts of love and knowing that we can learn to go within and meditate on three simple questions.

1. What do I need to know?

2. What do I need to learn?

3. What do I have to give?

These simple questions open such an infinite love, that we will know God for ourselves, not through some religion that seems to say "this is the only way and you're wrong if you don't follow this path!"

We can know God as love. This one revelation attracts such love to you that you will want to make love with passionate thoughts!

Know for yourself by affirming:

> *I am a channel for the divine intention to flow through my life from moment to moment and I see and think clearly in my mind and I give thanks.*

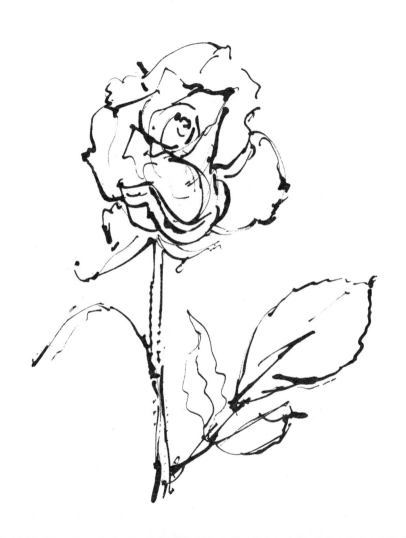

MEDITATION 34. AWARENESS

"If indeed you must be candid, be candid beautifully."

Kahlil Gibran

My friend Chelle Thompson, editor of www.inspirationline.com, passed this quote to me. Chelle imagined me saying what Kahlil wisely wrote above. Chelle, my editor, has a beautiful way of candidly making me aware of my blind spots; so lovingly that my child never feels scolded, even when I repeat myself in my writings.

Know for yourself and affirm:

As I become open to learning new ideas and skills I may make mistakes. People, who love me, gently point this out with beautiful love ... and my inner child feels loved. So I carry on wanting to learn.

And so it is.

MEDITATION 35. LIFE IN THE MIRROR

"Daily mirror work, saying a positive affirmation, tells me nearly instantly what beliefs are holding me back to loving myself."

Roger

When I looked into a mirror and said, "I love you" I wanted to scream "NO…NO…NO!" It seemed an absolute foreign and abusive language, saying such kind words to myself and especially into my own eyes. I had come to expect blame and criticism from me to me, and to begin with I looked anywhere but the mirror. The more I did mirror work the more I got to see what was holding me back from deserving that love from the power that made me. So start where you are willing. Know for yourself:

> *I let go of all need to criticise myself and when I do, I let this doubt dissolve with love and patience. And so it is.*

Remember you can be gentle and patient with yourself and do more daily mirror work saying, "I love and approve of you exactly as you are." Doubt may come up and say, "Stop kidding yourself."

Remember doubt has been there to protect you by saying a false truth "you can't love you, you're not good enough. " Just reassure doubt that this is an old belief and thank doubt for sharing then move on.

MEDITATION 36. ENERGY

*"Every thought and word is an affirmation; the more we choose
thoughts of love, joy, forgiveness and prosperity, the more our life
radiates a beauty that creates peace and harmony on this planet."*

Roger

Today I awoke with rain coming down on my bedroom window; my first thought,
'Oh it's wet." Then I changed the channel and tuned into choosing the thought,
'God is washing and replenishing the earth." As this happened I noticed how my
energy became stronger and I felt so close to living in the moment.

Know for yourself:

*As I choose a positive thought
I plant a seed in the garden of my
mind. It may feel untrue at first, yet
with patience and love it gradually
grows into divine love.
And I give thanks.*

MEDITATION 37. UNCONDITIONAL LOVE

"If a man does not keep pace with his companions, perhaps it is because he hears a different drummer. Let him step to the music which he hears, however measured and far away."

Henry David Thoreau

When we change and grow differently to what well-meaning people want us to do, who think they know what's best for us, we can feel a little confused or rejected and slightly crazy! Just now as I embark on a new career as a writer and publisher, I can sense disapproval from some good friends around me. Yet I have to know for myself:

I cannot afford the luxury of your negative thoughts about me and I don't need to justify myself to you. I send unconditional love to all family and friends as I follow the beat of the drum that comes from my heart and soul. And I give thanks.

Allow yourself to congratulate yourself for not conforming too old stereotypes, by saying *"I freely let all around me march to the beat of their own drum and I go forward with love and joy. And so it is."*

MEDITATION 38. CONNECTEDNESS

"What you are thinking and speaking right now is joining you to other souls on this planet. Who are you connecting to? People who blame and want revenge or the energy of love and forgiveness?"

Love and energy are interconnected. Love contains within it energy to unite human beings, because love alone joins all of us by what is deepest within ourselves. When I watch my 19-month-old grandson sleep, he lies totally open. His soul seems to open and is receptive to the love of God and attracts to himself such love from others around him. When I sleep at 56 years old, I curl up and sometimes think thoughts that don't invite divine energy to my soul.

We cannot see the wind, tide, and gravity, yet they are invisible laws of energy, which we are part of on this planet from moment to moment. So the more we think and speak love from a place of that loving baby soul, the more we attract intelligent love, compassionate unconditional love, and the more we harness love energy for God to heal, create, renew and bring universal love into visible existence.

Know for your soul:

I am open and receptive to abundant love that holds and heals every cell in the universe. Learning to love the miracle of my life radiates healing love for all on this planet and beyond.

MEDITATION 39. FEELING SAFE

"Now and then I go about pitying myself
and all the while my soul is being blown by
great winds across the sky."

A phrase from Ojibway Native American tribes

When I feel sorry for myself and I want to be important in a fearful way, I am learning to see my soul as blown across this great sky, it centres my thoughts to listen carefully and affirm the scared little child within. Know for yourself:

> *I am safe...*
> *it is only change...*
> *I love you and I am here for*
> *you, what can I do to help*
> *you feel safe?*

Then I listen with unconditional love. As I nurture myself, I find I truly value my life with all the twists and turns that made me who I am now.

MEDITATION 40. LOVE & WORK

*"When I work at something I love doing, like writing
and counselling I can at times devalue these gifts. Yet when
I work with love in my heart and soul, the hours
become like music to my soul."*

Roger

Working on raising our consciousness with passionate love is a labour worthy of divine love being magnetised to our souls.

Know gently in your conscious thought:

I am at one with creating work I love and this attracts more work and love that deepens my awareness and knowledge of being connected to all on this planet who think similar thoughts. And so it is.

MEDITATION 41. SELF-WORTH

"The essence of success for most people is a feeling of self-love, self-esteem, or self-worth.

Sanaya Roman & Duane Packer, Creating Money Keys to Abundance

Success comes from feeling successful in the present moment, not when you have reached a goal or have something you want. For me it is giving from abundance that comes from knowing my soul is connected to a power within that continually gives to me all good. I then see and know for myself that I am a channel of God's love. In affirming the following, watch for the resistance that is a wonderful insight into what you believe, that may delay your thinking and feeling good about yourself and giving your best to life. *"I am a success; I am uniquely intelligent. Whatever life gives me I will handle it! I congratulate myself often for going within to my higher self and radiating love and giving from abundance."*

Often we define success in material things… this is one dimension, yet without abundant love it can feel empty. Remember all the stars and planets are in the right order, affirm:

> *As I open my awareness to this source of love, my consciousness expands. I work and live in moment-to-moment experiences that seed and grow genuine self-esteem, self-worth and self-love by being a channel of divine love. And so it is.*

MEDITATION 42. GROW IN CONSCIOUSNESS

"As I grow in consciousness, a light shines an inner awareness into my soul. I know whom I have hurt and as my inner light becomes stronger, I learn to heal and forgive."

Roger

A warrior of light opens their soul to become consciously re-connected to the thought that life is not a game, it is a wonderful opportunity to give from abundance and that our source is within. Know for yourself:

I am at peace with each moment of my past, present and future and I love my thoughts for giving me life back abundantly. And I give thanks.

MEDITATION 43. CREATING A NEW CAPACITY TO LOVE

"I believe we are here to love ourselves and radiate this to the world. This capacity to love ourselves as a magnificent miracle of life has been well disguised by our past histories and the generations that have gone before. Experiencing for ourselves that we are a divine expression of love." Roger

Many of us think we have so many problems, yet when you get down to it, the most important area of our life is consciously knowing that we are loveable because we exist with a wonderful inner power that knows us through and through. This energy or power allows us to receive solutions to what we see as problems, which are actually lessons.

As we learn to love ourselves a little more each day, by going within and connecting to this power, we can love others and it is far easier for others to love us. This improves work, relationships, health, money, creativity and our joy in dancing intimately with life. Love of the real blueprint that we truly are attracts to us magnificent miracles of life. By contacting this blueprint, a prosperity of infinite intelligence radiates to all whom we meet. Know for yourself:

With the knowledge and awareness of making positive passionate thoughts to dissolve negative thoughts, I am clearer for the Power to give me a freedom to break out, to experience feeling connected to the abundant souls of love.

MEDITATION 44. ALLOWING

"The power within us is willing to give us our fondest dreams and enormous plenty instantaneously. The problem is that we are not open to receiving it."

Louise Hay, The Power is Within You

This morning I awoke at 2 am thinking about a letter that said "Unfortunately the buying department has decided not to stock your title LOVE THE MIRACLE YOU ARE at this time."

My immediate thought was a feeling of being kicked in the solar plexus; my unconscious mind said "I told you so … the book is not good enough." Doubt had a field day! The day before this I had just delivered the book to a supermarket chain, yet in my mind I immediately discounted that success. So a little forward and a little back … I needed to learn the lessons again. After meditating and just going within, this simple affirmation came: *"I allow and I am open and receptive to learning from this experience … and all good will flow from it."*

Did I believe it? Well a little bit and then I just repeated the above affirmation, until I got up and started typing and sending more good energy into marketing the book from my intuitive belief in the higher power that is there for me.

Remember when you get a setback, it is a time to learn, to just go within and listen gently and keep affirming:

I am safe even when I go a little backwards, all life loves and supports me and I am open to learning and to new insights.

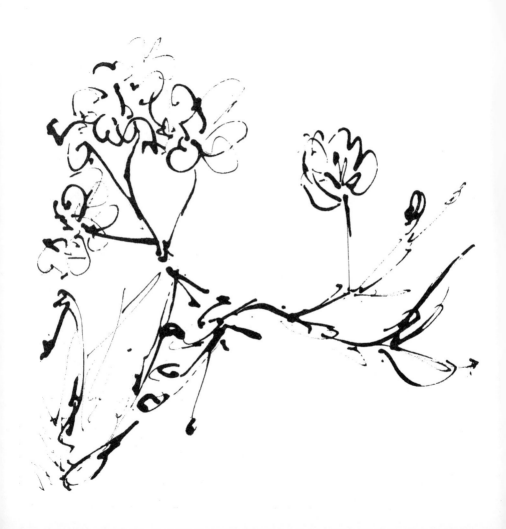

MEDITATION 45. DISSOLVING THE HURT

"Opening my arms to all good can bring up the opposite: I want to hide and scream out, "no, I am not good, I can't let all good in. I'll be found out as bad, wrong, stupid and everyone will laugh at me." This is simply the old message resurfacing from a hurt childhood." Roger

When I first tried positive affirmations, the words "I can't" came into the arena and I shrank away from any mirror. All I wanted to do was hide. If you find mirror work tough, be gentle with yourself and just know that you delay your prosperity by being so critical of YOU.

Dissolving all self-criticism seems extremely hard when our words so easily spill out with "I can't or "I won't, they don't work for me".

Just recently the past came back to me with a vengeance and I had to see what was my responsibility in making this happen. I became fearful and this sent me back into the past. When I am frightened I want to control everything by running away to bed, eating what I know I am going to regret and then beating myself up even more.

Yet I have learned to just repeat, from my loving inner parent:

I really, really love you; I know you're frightened, but I am here to help you so you will grow strong and true from this experience. Good will come out of it, for you are safe and divinely protected.

MEDITATION 46. ENERGY

"Connecting with energy is something humans have to be open to and talking about and expecting..."

James Redfield, The Celestine Prophecy

Today I walked into my favourite café and listened to the owner as she said, "I'd love my partner to read your book and he needs it! "I replied, "'Love The Miracle You Are' is a book that you pick up when you're open to the energy to change, when he's ready, he will."

Nobody will change and grow in consciousness, until THEY decide; you cannot force anybody to change; yet you can work on your own consciousness.

Know in your soul:

I now choose to take my power back by going within each day, affirming positive thoughts, that create experiences which release me from being responsible for everyone else's growth. And so it is.

MEDITATION 47. TRUST & PATIENCE

*"If you have been a very negative person who criticises yourself
and everyone else and sees life through very negative eyes, then it is
going to take time for you to start turning around and become loving..."*

Louise Hay, Heart Thoughts

Patience will be needed if critical parents have parented you; I found it so tough to listen carefully to my negative beliefs when I first tried to love myself. I just thought 'this is never going to work!' I never saw how impatient I was until I heard the affirmation:

> *The wisdom I seek is within me. I know there is plenty of time to love myself ... a little more each day.*
>
> *And so it is.*

Then, I also had to accept me just as I was, not perfect ... just me; with me being honest with myself in a gentle way a little more each day.

MEDITATION 48. LOVE & PASSION

"Surrender means the decision to stop fighting the world, and start loving it instead... liberation isn't about breaking out of anything; it's a gentle melting into who we really are."

Marianne Williamson, A Return To Love

When we surrender and just love from our conscious soul to our unconscious soul, it's like a light turns on inside our complete soul. Two halves come together and give up fighting, and then true passion with spontaneous intelligence is reborn. We gradually dissolve our addiction to control everything and everybody! Know in your heart the presence by daily affirming:

I choose passionate, loving thoughts and my unconscious mind loves them a little more each day and I truly leap with joy.

What comes back are miracles of life.

Healing and prosperity are an everyday occurrence in every seen and unseen area of my life. And I give thanks to the energy that guides me from deep within.

MEDITATION 49. FREE TO THINK

"Life flows with the freedom of unconditional love. This is the very essence of life."

Wayne Dyer, Manifest Your Destiny

Learning to think in your own mind and knowing God made you to choose your own thoughts is a freedom that is infinite. This I believe is a gift from the creator within each of us as human beings. Unconditional love allows you to think as you choose.

Know for yourself deep within your human soul:

My thoughts that I choose create my reality from moment to moment and I choose unconditional love.

And so it is.

MEDITATION 50. A CHANNEL FOR PASSION

"When you are ready your teacher will appear."

Anonymous

As we cease to be closed to learning, we change and we let go of control. We begin to feel "at one" with energy that reveals itself with teachers both human and "unseen," in nature, in books, in meditation, in passionate love making, in moments of ecstasy, in scripture, in the divine soul that speaks of many past lives and brings us to live in the now with an inner energy that radiates love. As this process evolves, we attract teachers who guide us with love at the centre of their hearts. We let go of being co-dependant about what others will think and say.

Stand with your arms wide open and declare with passion:

I am open and receptive to passionately making love to the miracle of life so that I can know and learn my purpose and meaning in this soul life.

AND I GIVE THANKS.

MEDITATION 51. HUMOUR HEALS

"Humour cuts oppressors down to size, takes their sting away, renders them powerless to destroy us. Don't give in to what diminishes you."

Joan Chittister, Songs of Joy

Often humour can help us heal the wounds of those who hurt us. As a counsellor try to help people laugh WITH their pain not just at it. Humour gives spirit and sustenance to the soul when a person has no other defence, it can give dignity when there is no other way. My wife Linda comes from a Jewish family and she read the following to me this morning from Joan Chittister's book.

"Jews delighted, for instance, in telling the story of the old man in top hat and phylacteries who appeared at the local Gestapo station. He was holding an ad in his hand that called for young, healthy Aryans to promise service to the Fuhrer. "What are you doing here?" the commandant asked the old Jew. "I am answering this ad," the old man said. "What?" the commandant asked incredulously. "That's ridiculous. You're not young." "No," the old man said, "I'm seventy-three." "And you're certainly not Aryan." "No," the old man said, "I'm Jewish-both sides." "And you're obviously not committed to serving the Fuhrer." "No," the old man said "I wouldn't do a single thing for that man." "Then why are you here?" The commandant insisted angrily." "Vell," the old Jew said … "I just came down to tell you that on me you shouldn't count."

Humour can help us regain our dignity by seeing life differently than we usually do. Know for yourself:

> *I use my humour wisely and I love to laugh at the paradoxes of life.*

MEDITATION 52. SPIRITUAL GROWTH

"I am not and you are not perfect ... we might become bores if we were!"

Roger

I see clearly that religion has often taken over as another parent control figure, often made up of individuals who don't love themselves from a place of deep self-respect. We have so often neglected the second part of Christ's commandment "Love thy neighbour as thyself." Consequently, religion is often NOT spiritual. Organised religion frequently undermines the human mind to think and see clearly. This of course, is not to deny your personal experience of religion and the way you practise your beliefs.

My spiritual journey has taken many twists and turns over 56 years. Often my spiritual growth comes when I have gone within and had some honest talks with myself and found a power and presence that directs me beyond old rigid beliefs. Spiritual growth for me is about being open and willing to learn from life and from books and tapes. It can come through a close friend whom we love dying, a personal crisis like a divorce, a physical dis-ease or when we truly walk alongside a soul who is going through tough times…or just listening to a skylark sing! It can happen when listening to some wonderful music or just being met by an inner whisper inside our souls. Laughing a great belly laugh and then crying with laughter.

Meditation, sitting quietly or just typing like now, is for me, spiritual, as I channel thoughts and feelings through this miracle mind, body and soul that I have been given to look after.

I notice from my "little life" that the more I step out of the victim role where I blame others and myself, a spiritual energy surges in every cell and organ of my body. The more I give myself permission to empower my life by choosing thoughts that forgive me and others, the less I stay trapped in self-righteousness. Then my spiritual path opens up without so much fear, criticism and GUILT. I love letting

o of guilt with love, because guilt doesn't help me in my spiritual journey. When
am made to feel guilty I ask myself "what is it that is manipulating me?" It can
e a person, a memory, a sermon, whatever, so I watch more carefully when I feel
nd think guilt thoughts.

So for me, I end these affirmations with:

*I love myself enough to let go of
all need to punish myself with beliefs
that no longer support me.*

*I love myself enough to forgive
myself and give myself over to a
higher consciousness that loves
me unconditionally.*

And I truly give thanks.

*"I affirm this little book will give you a desire to think and
feel passionately and that making love with passionate thoughts
really leads you to your highest good."*
My love, Roger.

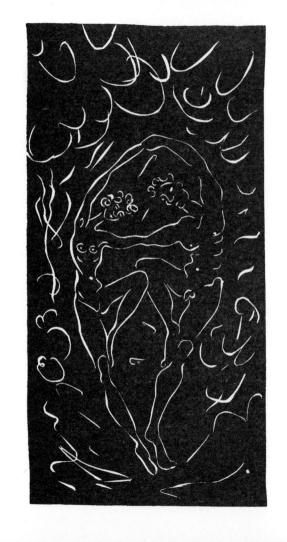

APPENDIX
<u>LITTLE GUIDELINES</u>

1. Place a Walkman by your bed and put in a positive tape by your favourite author. Put it on before you go to sleep and first thing in the morning. Then just notice the difference. You are reprogramming your subconscious mind and you may even fall asleep, but don't worry. As you connect more consciously to divine love, people, books and other resources will come exactly at the right time and perfect space sequence. Look on web site www.hayhouse.com for tapes and books, or go to www.soultalkstories.com and submit your soul story. Another wonderful website is www.inspirationline.com. Once you talk with passion and make love your goal, an infinite resource will come to you! Do explore my dear friend's website www.possibilitiesinaction.com and see what great coaching comes from a soul called Karin. My friend, Vidya, is a talented website designer whom you may visit at: www.webwisesage.com

2. The biggest lie we have been told is: "not to love ourselves because we are sinful and unworthy," yet Christ DID mention "… love thy neighbour as thyself." *You are worthy of love from the maker that made you, go within and listen and lovingly forgive YOU. Talk to this power with passionate loving thoughts. And so it is.*

3. "DO IT NOW!" On waking, drink a cup of warm boiled water and let your body re-hydrate. Then sit and meditate quietly. Listen carefully. Ask simple questions like: *What do you want me to know? What do you want me to learn?* Slow the thoughts and see what comes during the day. A lovely book to dip into is: "Love The Miracle You Are" by me, Roger King.

4. Body exercise. When I have found myself frightened by life, I realise I have been making MYSELF fearful; so I know it's time to use my energy by letting my

body move vigorously. Personally, I love the gym and sometimes I put a tape on and then I am exercising mind and soul AND body. Vary your exercise … run, walk, swim, cycle, and dance and move your body.

5. Keep uppermost in your mind that loving and forgiving thoughts release your blocked energy.*"I release with love all who criticize me including myself."*

6. Over 30 years of sitting opposite people who are hurting, the thing that I get most criticised for is offering "too much" hope and "positive thought" that their life can change and grow. When people say, "I hate myself," I ask them to shift their focus and develop a different outcome. I sometimes catch their dis-ease and believe them; then I shake myself free and give them my best, by reminding them that they truly will achieve whatever they desire.Memorize Italian painter, architect and poet Michelangelo's wise words:*"The greatest danger for most of us is not that our aim is too high and we miss it, but that it is too low and we achieve it."*

7. Remember, as you love your higher self (the part of you that has love at the very core of you), the more you will grow in confidence. Your greater confidence diminishes the need for conditional approval. A strange paradox will become true, this is: the more you love the power within you and know it as abundant love, the less you will need approval from those who don't have your highest interests at heart. Affirm: *"I release with forgiveness and love any warped or obsessive need for others' approval of me. I now attract people who love to grow in consciousness and we create circles of love in this life. And so it is."*

Thank you for yourself, giving you back to you, the miracle blue print of you.

My love,

Roger.

(Do give feedback and submit your soul story on our website www.soultalkstories.com)

MAKING LOVE WITH PASSIONATE DRAWINGS

"When Rog said he would like to use some of my drawings in this book I was delighted. So included are a selection of a few images that hold for me particular elements of passionate living. I have also included some words which may or may not be helpful for the viewer. My hope is that these too may enhance your experience of passionate Life."

CHOICES

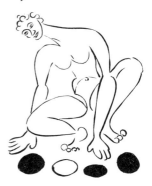

Originally inspired by an image from the Motherpeace pack which shows a woman pondering her cards/ life choice/opportunities. She is still, reflective, meditative. The need is to be quiet, solitary, alone as we make our own decisions and choices.

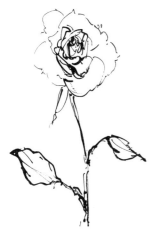

ROSE

The rose has long been a symbol of beauty, romance, love and passion. The fragile beauty of the petals and the piercing thorns represent both the pain and joy of our love and passion. You cannot have the bloom without the thorns. As the tightly packed bud unfurls so our heart centre opens and closes and opens again. It felt necessary to have the rose included in MLWPT.

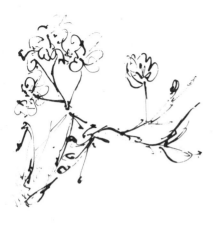

CHERRY BLOSSOM

Last week the Cherry trees broke into the pink splendour of their blossoming. Days later they had already began dropping their petals confetti- like into pools under the trees. So transient, so beautiful, how to impress their beauty within our minds to hold onto and be nourished by throughout the year?

BRIDAL SUITE

Is about unity and oneness, a celebration of intimacy in relationships and the joy of 'marriage' meaning here the celebration of love between man and woman, the masculine and the feminine, joining in perfect balance and harmony creating together the balanced whole. Created from many hours spent watching and drawing dancers coupled with the beauty of the May blossom which overhangs a local bridal way the image was born and I discovered there was a romantic inside of me.

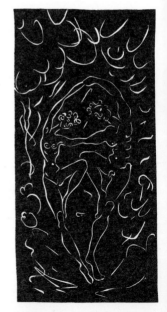